The Art of Weight Reduction

The Art of Weight Reduction

R.C. COOLEY

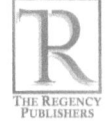
THE REGENCY PUBLISHERS

Copyright © 2022 by R.C. Cooley.

All rights reserved. No part of this book may be reproduced in any form or by any electronic or mechanical means, including information storage and retrieval systems, without permission in writing from the author and publisher, except by reviewers, who may quote brief passages in a review.

ISBN: 978-1-960113-30-6 (Paperback Edition)
ISBN: 978-1-960113-31-3 (Hardcover Edition)
ISBN: 978-1-960113-29-0 (E-book Edition)

Book Ordering Information

The Regency Publishers, US
521 5th Ave 17th floor NY, NY10175
Phone Number: (315)537-3088 ext 1007
Email: info@theregencypublishers.com
www.theregencypublishers.com

Printed in the United States of America

Contents

Book Summary ix
Introduction xi
Purpose of book xiii
Chapter 1 The Igen Process, A must-have skill for the 20th
  Century 1
Chapter 2 Three Biological Principles Underlying the Igen
  Process 2
Chapter 3 A Paradigm Shift 4
Chapter 4 Features of the Igen Process: 6
Chapter 5 Origins of our weight epidemic 7
    Food Industry 7
    Hyperpalatable foods 7
    High Fructose corn syrup 8
    Weight Loss industry 8
Chapter 6 What is Obesity? 10
    FTO, the hunger gene. 11
Chapter 7 Overeating, an internal problem 13
    Who is responsible? 14
Chapter 8 We're at a Crossroads 16
Chapter 9 Why does the Igen Process work? 18
    Overnight weight loss - The big Fast 18
    Data gathering by student 20
    Food logs 20

Weight Log	21
Discussion	21
Chapter 10 Online class	22
A Do-It-Yourself 3 step solution:	23
Reading 1 Weight Reduction-The Loneliest Task	24
Reading 2 Weight Reduction as an Art Form	26
Reading 3 Excess Weight Shortens Lifespans	28
Emotional suffering	28
Reading 4 Physical Complications of Excess Weight	30
Reading 5 Willpower Misunderstood	31
Weight loss means NO	33
Head for your ideal weight and be happy	33
Reading 6 The Allure of Fat, Sugar and Salt	35
Fat benefits	36
Sugar benefits	36
Salt benefits:	37
Reading 7 Overeating, a Genetic Drive to Survive	38
Our Lizard Brain	38
Modern Times	39
It's in The Genes	39
Reading 8 Automatic Eating	41
Why Do We Eat?	41
Most eating is subconscious behavior	41
Hunger has nothing to do with it	42
Food, a feel-good source	42
So, What Can Be Done?	43
Reading 9 The Mathematics of Weight Gain and Weight Loss	44
What you eat counts	44
Not rocket science	45

Reading 10 The Use of Imagery and Affirmations 46
    What is imagery? 47
    What is an affirmation? 47
    Application of imagery and affirmation. 47

Reading 11 Becoming an Expert 49
    Expert secrets 49
    Making new behavior automatic 50

Reading 12 Food Combinations That Affect Your Metabolic Rate 51
    What is metabolism? 51
    How your diet can speed up your metabolism 52

Reading 13 Malleability of Food Preferences 53
    Childhood has a big influence in food preferences 54

Reading 14 How to Deal with Cravings 56
    Trick your brain 57
    Why Do We Crave Sugar? 57
    Strategies to Break the Craving Cycle 58

Reading 15 Setting up your own Igen Process center: 60

Biography 61

Book Summary

This book is designed to cut through the confusion and uncertainty of obesity and to serve as an instructional guide to anyone who wants to reduce their weight. The process described in this book is rooted in measurement and observation and is effective regardless of eating preferences or activity levels. In other words, it doesn't require exercise or changing the type of foods you eat. The readings are also designed to leave the user with the tools and mindset to maintain their ideal weight permanently once they get there. We spend 62 billion dollars every year in this country for weight loss products and services when the solution is literally in our hands. This book describes the Igen Process, its biological underpinnings, and how to engage in the process. This book also serves as a companion to the online class which walks you week after week, and month after month, to a gradual but permanent reduction in your weight. Understanding our body, our mid-brain, our food environment, and how they interact, gives us the necessary insight to intervene and return to our ideal weight.

Introduction

Since I wrote my first book. The Art of Losing Weight, the obesity epidemic has been steadily increasing both in the US and worldwide, especially in developing nations. It seems that industrialization and something innately human are at the root of this phenomenon that diminishes our quality of life and threatens our very existence.

If there has ever been an existential crisis for the human species it is now. We ingest fat, sugar, and salt, in quantities that make them toxic. They either clog our arteries, scar them from the inside or perturb our intestinal flora and cause digestive problems. We distort our body shape with excessive fat accumulation. It's maddeningly frustrating that we still freely and willingly engage in behaviors that are detrimental to our wellbeing. We are not a world of masochists so why do we do it? Simple!

We are directed by genetic blueprints embedded in our midbrain! And in the absence of knowledge of how these blueprints work and what they cause, we trust our brain when it tells us we are hungry. Willpower by itself cannot stand up to biology. And make no mistake; weight reduction is a biological challenge.

It's time that everyone has a roadmap to weight reduction. This book will help the reader with the process of developing this roadmap as we gradually understand the general dynamics of obesity and begin to understand our own personal dynamics with respect to eating. For children, who are also at risk, it is their caregivers who have the responsibility to develop the ability to protect them from excess weight taking hold.

It's time to ask why, after 50 years of sounding the alarm, obesity is still rampant and impacting our health negatively. It continues to diminish our quality of life and drive up our already soaring healthcare costs.

We want to eliminate obesity but we keep flooding our food supply with sugars, fats and salts. Our weight is out of control because we don't know much about the dynamics of excess weight or how our behavior interacts with these dynamics. The other reason weight is out of control is the reticence by both practitioners and patients to delve too deep into such a personal and private matter as eating. We consider eating to be one of the last frontiers of personal freedom and we resist being deprived of pleasure and comfort giving foods we are used to.

However, apart from our own behavior, a huge factor in our country's headlong spiral into obesity are two industries; the food industry and the weight loss industry. The food industry floods our food supply with products spiked with pleasure-giving sugars, fats, and salts. These products are designed to hijack our brain's attention and to elicit a desire to eat.

The weight loss industry falls short by only focusing on burning calories by using equipment and activities. Ironically, this is something that the body already does extremely well, as we shall see later.

This fat burning strategy ignores the other side of the obesity equation which is preventing the unregulated accumulation and buildup of fat.

Purpose of book

The purpose of this book is to cut through the confusion and misunderstanding about obesity and weight reduction by introducing The Igen Process. The book can also serve as an instruction manual for anyone who wants to return to their ideal weight, or guide others, including pets, to their ideal weight.

This process is rooted in measurement and observation and is effective regardless of eating preferences or activity levels. Engage the Igen Process and I promise you will return to your ideal weight and acquire the ability to guide others to their desired weight.

Let me reiterate the purpose of the Igen Process; to reduce anyone's weight by focusing on the only behavior that increases weight; overeating. While weight reduction is a move towards health, achieving health is a more intimate and personal task that involves looking deeper into changes in different areas. I believe that engaging in physical activity and proper nutrition are vital to our health and we encourage everyone to do so. However, the success of our weight reduction program lies in the student's engagement with the Igen Process.

Chapter 1

The Igen Process, A must-have skill for the 20th Century

The Igen Process is a series of steps taken with an instructor that measure amounts and types of foods eaten, and your weight at different times. With this information we can structure an ongoing plan to begin your permanent weight reduction.

The Igen Process has many moving parts in that it measures and observes physiology, physical responses, weight, time, type and amounts of foods, etc. in order to have the data needed to proceed with your managed weight reduction.

But just like you can drive your car without knowing what is happening under the hood, you can engage in the Igen Process, without initially understanding the process. It will make no difference in your progress. Your progress is assured when you engage in the process.

The Igen Process is primarily learned through experiencing it and seeing its results in real time. This experience can be in person, or in an online class. As you engage in the Igen Process and observe, analyze, and discuss the results with your instructor, your understanding will catch up.

Chapter 2

Three Biological Principles Underlying the Igen Process

#1) The only source of energy for our body is food. Being lazy or a couch potato does not increase your weight, nor is avoiding exercise a factor in gaining weight.

#2) Weight is a dynamic process, it is never stable. It rises sharply when you eat and it goes down minute after minute hour after hour, when you are not eating and it rises sharply when you eat again.

#3) Any disruption to our food supply triggers an extreme physical and mental distress response. Among other energy conserving responses, it slows down your metabolism in order to retard the depletion of energy. This makes it very difficult to continue reducing your weight.

The activities in the Igen Process are designed to work with these three principles and not against them.

The Igen Process is basically a reverse engineering of your path to obesity. Thus we need to know where you are on this path by identifying how, when, and where you gain weight, and then devising behavioral strategies to reverse these patterns.

Weight is a side effect of the amount of food we eat. And everyone's current weight is a reflection of the amount of food they eat. The ultimate goal of the Igen Process is to have you eat the amount of food your body requires to be at your ideal weight. However, our body cannot tolerate a continuous reduction so it quickly reaches a plateau and stops losing weight.

That's why it is very difficult to reduce your weight by 30 pounds, but not that difficult to reduce your weight by 3 pounds, 10 times. Everyone knows how to lose weight. What we don't know is how to keep it off. This is the missing piece that The Igen Process supplies through the food and weight log measurements and analysis.

The Igen Process is not a quick fix, but it is a permanent fix. The sequence of a weight loss phase followed by a maintenance phase is crucial in being able to manage your weight reduction. It gives your metabolism time to adjust to the reduced amount of food, and the new lower weight.

The strategic review of your data and the planning with your instructor helps you navigate the external influences in the environment that facilitate and encourage eating, and the internal physiological and psychological forces designed to prevent you from starving. And since any significant weight loss is interpreted by our brain as imminent starvation, it immediately deploys and elicits these forces to prevent further loss.

The Igen Process is a thorough accounting of the food we eat, our weight at specific points in time, and an analysis of the correlation between what you eat and how much you weigh. This analysis yields information for the planning sessions with your instructor and is the reason that delivering the Igen Process through a class format with regular meeting intervals is most effective.

Chapter 3

A Paradigm Shift

How do I lose weight? The answer to this question is complex since it has hundreds of answers! Running, walking, dancing, jumping, pushups, bicycling, hiking, joining a gym or exercise group etc., are all ways of burning calories. Not eating refined flour, not drinking fruit juices, or sugary drinks, eating small portions, are ways to reduce the acquisition of calories.

When you attempt to lose weight with these strategies, it's a big deal. You have to buy memberships, travel to the gym, learn equipment uses, buy appropriate clothes, etc. And you engage in these activities because your purpose is to burn more calories to lose weight. However, this complex problem becomes a simple problem when we shift our focus and instead ask, How do I gain weight? And since the only activity that produces weight gain is eating, all we have to do is focus on our eating behavior which is totally under our control.

This shift away from seeking weight loss, towards identifying how we gain weight will yield more useful answers for our weight reduction plans.

While this paradigm shift may seem to be at first glance merely a semantic sleight of hand, the shift moves 'losing weight' away from being the goal, to being a benchmark in the process. Also, equipping yourself with the knowledge of how you use food to gain weight will allow you to customize an approach that will fit no one else but you. It is also the most humane way because it works within your personal tolerance levels for food deprivation.

The Igen Process is a coherent and transparent approach to weight reduction, that engages the individual on the one thing that leads to obesity, their eating behavior, not their food. This paradigm shift isn't merely a play on words, it also changes the focus of our activities.

The activities we traditionally engage in to lose weight are the following: **Calorie burning.** We raise our metabolic rate through various kinds of physical activity to burn a higher amount of calories. **Eating differently.** We change what and how much we eat to lower our calorie intake. **Bariatric surgery.** A procedure that helps you eat less by removing or stapling portions of your stomach or intestine.

The behaviors we engage in the Igen Process to identify weight gain are the following: **Food monitoring.** Being aware of what you eat, and **Eating less** which means adopting a mindset of looking for opportunities to eat less. (Exercise and healthy nutrition have nothing to do with weight gain thus they are not within the scope of our activities).

Chapter 4

Features of the Igen Process:

We have redefined the problem away from complexity and towards simplicity by asking How do I gain weight, instead of How do I lose weight? The simplicity comes from the fact that we have to attend to only one behavior to answer this question i.e. eating.

We also have genetics on our side because we can modify the behavior of the gene responsible for our hunger or desire for food.

And we also have the knowledge of physiological and psychological barriers to our weight reduction that we can prepare for, and anticipate.

And finally we have a step by step sequenced process that will guide you to your ideal weight by analyzing the data that you provide and an instructor to help you craft real time strategies and interventions for immediate application.

CHAPTER 5

Origins of our weight epidemic

Food Industry

The food industry has been a huge influence in our collective health decline. They accidentally stumbled onto the FTO gene's mission to seek out opportunities to eat and give us pleasure, and its preference for dense calorie foods. Understanding that our brain prefers dense calorie offerings, the food industry responded by creating a new category of food that satisfies the brain's preference for dense calorie foods.

Hyperpalatable foods

These are products that pack high amounts of fat, salt, or sugar in their composition. The purpose is to make them calorie dense so the brain will prefer it over other choices. In a sense, hijacking the brain away from its less caloric choices. There is nothing in the natural world that by volume packs the calories of a hamburger or a milkshake.

One of the first popular hyperpalatable creations is the variety of soft drinks. Each 12 oz. can contains approximately 10 teaspoons of sugar each. A decision by Coca Cola a few years back, to increase their presence in Mexico, began by putting their product in the most remote villages where the only shiny object was the Coke dispenser. A few years later this had the effect of propelling Mexico to surpass the United States' leading position in obesity.

Currently in the U.S. research has shown that soft drink beverages account for 16% of the US obesity statistics.

High Fructose corn syrup

The food industry also created a new type of sugar called High Fructose Corn Syrup which is a combination of fructose and glucose. The glucose is processed at the cellular level throughout the body. However, fructose in excess amounts is a health hazard because it is processed in the liver into fats where they can build up and enter the bloodstream causing obesity, hypertension, insulin resistance and type II diabetes.

The use of this product in our food supply since the 1970's has increased the average amount of sugar consumed by each person per year from 15 pounds in the 1950's to 90 pounds in 2018.

Weight Loss industry

Weight loss has been an elusive goal for millions of people. We are told that exercising and eating healthy will solve our weight problems. Last year, 60 billion dollars were spent on weight loss products and services, yet, this year 85% of the US population is either overweight or obese.

Even more troubling are statistics that show this rise in our obesity index has happened every single year for the last 50 years. It has never decreased or even remained stable from one year to the next. This is a clear indication that our obesity epidemic is out of control. The health professions have never been able to guide us to reduced weights with their products.

In 2021, 27% of our children fell into the obese category. If these children do nothing now, they will face a lifetime of medical issues.

Chapter 6

What is Obesity?

Obesity is the result of a genetic bias all humans have to accumulate fuel in the form of fat. It affects every individual and has led millions to chronic weight gain over the years. One of the results of this weight gain is that the external appearance of our body changes shape as the accumulation increases year after year.

To see if you are under the influence of this bias, read each statement to see how many you are in agreement with.

1) I have lost weight and then regained it.
2) I have tried to lose weight more than once.
3) I am heavier today than a year ago.
4) There are foods I can't do without.

If you agree with two or more of these statements, you need to rethink your strategy or efforts to lose weight because you may be under the influence of an overactive FTO gene.

Obesity is one of the most insidious threats to our collective wellbeing. For most, excess weight is an aesthetical problem because it changes our body by depositing the additional fat it is accumulating on a daily basis, at different points on our body. The pattern of distribution is genetically dictated and usually comes off in the reverse order that it was accumulated.

If the fat is stored on our back, shoulders, or neck our appearance will be top heavy. If it's stored on our buttocks, legs, or thighs, our appearance will be bottom heavy. When it's stored on the hips and abdomen, our appearance will be round. However, this fat around the middle may also be signaling a more dangerous condition that happens when fat settles on the internal organs as opposed to under the skin giving the person a pregnant look. This visceral fat is dangerous because the organ reacts to the fat as foreign matter and develops inflammation that may interfere with its function. Obesity also aggravates many other conditions, and afflictions people may already be battling.

FTO, the hunger gene.

The gene responsible for this bias toward the unregulated accumulation of fat, is the FTO gene. This gene is constantly alert to the presence of food in its environment as it fulfills its primary mission to accumulate fuel for the organism. When it detects food through our senses, it will activate and begin its foraging behavior, which is to seek out opportunities to eat anywhere in its vicinity or environment.

This gene emerged 17 million years ago. We see the extreme effects of this accumulation in the morbidly obese, who can reach weights of 700 plus pounds. Most people will take action earlier and much before their ability to move is compromised, but it's the same mechanism that drives the overeating in all of us.

This gene is located in the brain's Limbic System where many life sustaining automatic functions reside such as breathing, heartbeat, digestion, etc. It is not surprising that the urge to eat has a large automatic component to it.

This particular type of gene is called an expressive gene, and it "suggests" to the individual a course of action. The suggestions from the FTO gene entail some type of eating activity. However, we have the ability to ignore this message, if we know and understand that its origin is not real hunger but comes from the influence of the FTO gene. on its mission to accumulate fuel.

This gene is stimulated to eat by seeing, smelling, tasting, and even remembering food. Thus, eating stimulates the gene to keep us eating until we physically can't fit any more food into our stomach and stop. The stimulation of this gene also comes from advertising and marketing sources and is a relentless 24/7 a barrage of ads touting newer, improved, and tastier compositions.

These marketing efforts saturate our environment with sugary and fatty snacks from gas stations to auto supply stores in addition to fast food outlets and supermarkets. All have candies or snacks at their checkout counters. Those who permit this gene's influence to overrule their cerebral cortex at the check out lanes, will purchase these products as a habit and progressively accumulate fat until they are in the obese category.

Simply stated, fat is the only substance that will provide the energy our body needs to carry out its functions, and the only way we get fat is through our diet.

The body is a complex machine that will extract nutrients from carnivorous or vegetarian diets and convert it to fat. It accumulates this new fat in specialized fat storage cells. It is when this accumulation becomes excessive that we define it as obesity. Between The "push" of the food industry and the "pull" of the FTO gene, chronic weight gain has emerged as a looming threat on the horizon of the human species and it has been consistently herding us all towards obesity.

Chapter 7

Overeating, an internal problem

A strict definition of overeating is: the consumption of all food that contributes to keep us away from our ideal weight. A looser definition is: the mechanism that leads us slowly and surely to chronic weight gain which eventually results in obesity. The body expends energy 24/7 and eats to replace the expended energy. Overeating is when the consumption of food exceeds the calories that were expended leaving us with a net gain of calories the following day in the form of fat.

Obesity starts when by overeating we inadvertently add a few pounds and then few more, until we begin noticing blouses, shirts, pants, and belts begin to tighten on us. Unfortunately, after we try to lose weight and can't, we just go out and buy a larger size. This will go on for the rest of our life unless we recognize what is happening and take simple but consistent action.

The extra few pounds slipped in unnoticed because it happens very gradually through overeating. If you overeat and increase your weight one quarter ounce daily, it will be completely unnoticed. The math tells us that in 4 days your total weight increased by 1 ounce. Again, too small to be noticed. However, this rate of growth will roughly add about 5 pounds per year. It is this constant gain that can be easily tracked and addressed in real time through the Igen Process.

In 2013 the American Medical Association classified obesity as a disease. Not so much for its pathology, but rather for its positive correlation with so many diseases and conditions. It's my hope that the message from the AMA in classifying it as a disease is to encourage the healing profession to treat excess weight. The standard approach to treating obesity is to ask the patient to lose weight by attending an exercise class and/or a nutrition class and to report back in a few months. During those 2 or 3 months, because he's not aware, the client is ambushed again and again by biological and physiological mechanisms in place to protect our body against any significant weight reduction.

The obesity problem has grown so large and is so intractable that most overweight persons make peace with their excess weight, accept it as permanent, and use fashion and fabric to disguise or conceal their girth. However, there is a price to pay. The average lifespan of newer generations is expected to be shorter than previous ones. Diet-based afflictions and conditions like diabetes, hypertension, coronary heart disease, diverticulosis, etc., are on the rise, spurred on by our consumption of products loaded with fats, sugars and salts, and served in larger and larger sizes.

This paints a grim picture making obesity likely and shorter lifespans probable for these coming generations. Unfortunately, not only is there no trend reversal in sight, but many of these conditions are now appearing earlier in the lives of children.

Who is responsible?

When we don't understand the dynamics of excess weight, we can truly say that obesity is not our fault. However, when we understand the causes and factors surrounding excess weight and how our actions propel us towards obesity, and then we fail to act, the responsibility for our obesity becomes ours. We eat guided by our food preferences and eating patterns, thus, what we eat, how much we eat, where we eat, when we eat and even why we eat are as unique to each individual as their thumbprint.

Whether you grew up eating salads, soups, meats and fruits, or eating pizza, hamburgers, lasagna and spaghetti, will make a difference in your weight gain over time. However, because eating is so personal and mostly private, you are the only one who can make any changes. Therefore, you must consciously know about your preferences and habits and how they influence your weight.

Chapter 8

We're at a Crossroads

We are at a critical moment in our evolution as a species. The existential question for our times is, Will we as a society, be able to pull out of this nosedive into obesity? Will we grasp the concept of a "rogue gene" whose survival value is no longer needed, but that continues to exert its influence on our behavior, now to the detriment of our health?

Eventually evolution will dictate a mutation to restructure our behavioral repertoire to reflect the abundance of food in our environment. However, we can't wait thousands of years for that to happen. Till then, to counteract its influence we have created a deliberate intervention format in the form of the Igen Process, to consciously approve or deny every intention of our brain to eat. This involves creating and adopting a mindset to successfully engage the Igen Process and understand your weight buildup.

This mindset must be present always because it reminds us to make choices every time we are face to face with food. The strength of the Igen Process lies in the methodical manner it identifies and deflects urges and ingrained habits with purposeful action. A focus on exercise and healthy nutrition confuses the weight reduction issue. The Igen Process deals only with weight reduction and that means dealing with amounts, not types of food.

The simplicity of the approach to reduce your weight belies the complex and intense nature of our body's formidable physiological and psychological defenses designed to resist any significant weight loss.

Chapter 9

Why does the Igen Process work?

Because it focuses on the root cause of obesity which is our own behavior! Our body is a formidable calorie burning machine that runs 24/7, even when we sleep. It does not need our help to burn calories! In fact, in the time between your last meal of the day and your first meal in the morning, as you were sleeping your body lost between 1 and 3 pounds.

Understanding the mechanisms of excess weight and your own personal dynamics will let you craft a customized strategy that takes your lifestyle into account. This process is a simple systematic approach to eating less. It consists of a reduction phase and a maintenance phase. Through this process, you take direct control of your weight since you are the only one that can put food in your mouth. The goal is to reach your ideal weight as per the BMI chart.

Overnight weight loss - The big Fast

Fasting is defined as the state of needing fuel without nutrients in our stomach. The body then uses the accumulated fuel to power its physiological functions. Weight lost during sleep is a measure of your body's resting metabolic rate. It is also a permanent loss. Which means that to get this weight back you need to eat.

We said peviously that our body is an amazing fat burning machine.

Would you believe that our body loses the equivalent of its total body weight every 4 to 5 weeks. Let's do the math. If you lose 1.5 pounds overnight (a modest reduction for 8 hours sleep), you will lose 4.5 pounds in 24 hours. In ten days you will lose 45 pounds. In 30 days you will lose 135 pounds. The reason we don't notice this weight loss is because we have also had 90 meals plus snacks throughout these 30 days.

You can see the number of calories being spent by your body per day is very large. And the beauty of it is that the only way the body replaces these calories is through eating. The reason for this massive burning of calories is that once your last meal of the night is digested, the only source of fuel to keep your heart beating, your lungs contracting, your brain thinking, and your digestive process in action, is your stored body fat. And each calorie that you burn to keep your metabolism running has a corresponding amount of fat that disappears from your body in the form of weight. This is permanent weight loss! If you don't replace it, it doesn't come back.

Your personal efforts to lose weight will always be minimal in comparison to the ongoing energy demands of your body. However, be aware that when you are overweight, losing weight will evoke a strong response from your body and mind to keep you at the same weight. How you deal with these resistance responses will determine if they pose a serious threat to your weight reduction goals or not. Knowing and expecting the resistance will prepare you to deal with it as it happens. However, if you don't recognize it as coming from within you, it will most likely sabotage your efforts.

Data gathering by student

This feature sets us apart from most weight reduction programs. We gather weight data both in the morning and in the evening. In the Igen Process your evening weight is a marker that helps you reach your ideal weight by monitoring your weight gain when it counts, during the day when your foraging behavior is active and you can do something about it.

Once you weigh yourself in the morning, there is nothing you can do about your weight. Not so when you monitor your evening weight. Once you know your overnight weight loss you can factor it in to predict your morning weight. We also gather food data whenever you eat anything or drink anything, except water and black coffee. We then take these two measurements and analyze them to draw conclusions about your weight gain. We can see patterns of eating, amounts of carbs, proteins, etc. and we see if they line up with your goals. If your night/morning weight differential is small, it indicates a slow metabolism. We look at the food log to see why. Maybe you are eating too many carbs in the evening which slows down your metabolism. Without these data measurements we are flying blind.

Food logs

This log records the time you ate, where you ate, what you ate, how much or how many you ate, and why. The purpose is to raise an awareness of our eating behavior. All food sources; home, coffee shop, restaurant, corner market, lunch room need to be identified. Think of it as mapping out the threats in your environment. Habits and eating patterns are outed and scrutinized for their positive or negative influence towards your weight reduction. The food log also identifies your food preferences and how they influence your metabolism.

Weight Log

This log records your morning and evening weights to confirm that the Igen Process is on track. It can also measure the strength of your metabolism. When this log is correlated with the Food log, we can see results, make projections and develop strategies going forward. It also validates the process and your experience as you see the correlation between the food log and the weight log and the effect on your progress. It also provides us with the data that tells us when to move to the next phase of the process

Discussion

The data from these measurements is analyzed and discussed with your instructor in order to continue, modify, or change the planned strategy or strategies. We do an analysis of carbs, fats, and vegetables from the food log, and see how they correlate to the weight log. Trends and patterns in our eating behavior are discussed, as well as any modifications to our overall strategic plan.

Chapter 10

Online class

Through the online class, we will guide you to your ideal weight day after day, and week after week until you reach your goal. We do this without requiring you to exercise or abstain from eating things that you like or are used to. In turn, you agree to write down everything you eat, log your weight twice a day, and meet regularly with your instructor to analyze the data, and discuss your next steps.

As I see it, we have three problems:

1. - An external problem that distorts our body and lowers our quality of life, i.e. obesity. The solution here is to reduce the rate of accumulation.
2. - An internal problem that propels us consistently towards excess weight and obesity, i.e. overeating. The solution is to recognize the origin of these desires.
3. - A social problem that infuses large amounts of sugar, fats, and salts into our food supply. The solution here is for you to become an expert on your own nutrition.

A Do-It-Yourself 3 step solution:

1) Reduce your food intake consistently for any amount of time.
2) Notice when you reach a plateau
3) Maintain the same amount of food intake for approximately four weeks until your metabolism stabilizes. Repeat the 3 steps again. If you completed the previous cycle, you should now be at a lower weight.

The rest of this book will present foundational concepts that will provide you the basis to make this paradigm shift, where the focus is weight gain reversal, and the goal is to eat less in a planned manner until you are eating for the body you want.

Reading 1

Weight Reduction-The Loneliest Task

During the 50's and 60's when excess weight began to emerge among the population, we failed to recognize it as a public health issue. Through our inaction, we allowed private industry to address our excess weight problem. We went along and listened to their experts and tried their solutions. We ate low fat versions of most products without knowing that the fat being removed was replaced with sugar. We tried exercise and fitness programs, health food, and other chemical compositions from the pharmaceutical industry claiming to burn our fat off or block it from accumulating. We eat healthy food because we're told it will help us lose weight. To date, many believe the additives in our food and in the food supply of the animals we eat are implicated in our excess weight epidemic. We even let surgeons cut, staple or tie parts of our organs as a solution.

We have trusted all the above because we don't know anything else. Our weight loss strategies, efforts, goals and choices have been thought out for us. We are bombarded by a multitude of methods to lose weight, many that contradict each other. We're told to cut carbs, to cut fat, do vigorous exercise, do moderate exercise, to eat portions, to eat more often, etc. The result is a confusing array of products and methods. Ironically, one of the most extreme methods on the scene, bariatric surgery is useless if the person does not permanently reduce their consumption of food after the surgery. It is a truism that unrestrained eating will doom any exercise or nutritional approach, including bariatric surgery.

Furthermore, most traditional weight loss programs don't address weight loss directly. Their primary purpose is to sell a product or process that they believe will cause weight loss. Then they cross their fingers and hope you can make it work! If it does work, the program takes credit, if it doesn't work, then it's your fault. And how convoluted is it, that now even fast food outlets, restaurants and soft drink conglomerates have entered the weight loss industry to attract more clientele. Menus that have "healthy alternatives" or that show meal calorie counts do so to attract those concerned with their weight. Conveying in fact that they know you have a problem and they can help you. Soft drink makers are marketing smaller size containers also to help you lower your sugar intake.

Among this vast array of methods and products aimed at weight loss we have yet to come up with a "magic bullet". Since the 50's the general population weight index has risen year after year. We are not alone, excess weight is now the norm in most developed nations. Although fitness and nutritional approaches work for some, they have been a spectacular failure amongst the general population.

Reading 2

Weight Reduction as an Art Form

The American Heritage College Dictionary defines art as "human effort to imitate, supplement, alter or counteract the work of nature" It further defines it as "the conscious production or arrangement of elements in a manner that affects the senses" Chronic weight gain is a natural process mediated by brain structures to enhance the survival of our species by storing fuel as body fat. This is also the process underlying the obesity crisis that has been ravaging the industrialized world.

To counteract this natural process, we organize and arrange the following elements; What we eat, how much we eat, where we eat and at what time we eat. We learn how to detect the origin of our desire to eat as either a physiological need or a comfort need. And just as a sculptor needs to know marble composition, chiseling tools, angles etc. A person engaged in losing weight needs to know about external influences like advertising, marketing, and food composition. They should also be aware of internal influences like the FTO gene's influence, their metabolism, and the cerebral cortex.

The art lies in creating a lifestyle where your routine, activities, habits, and food preferences are arranged and manipulated in order to line up and support your weight reduction goals. This process is different for every person because eating patterns are as individual as fingerprints. Even those who live together and eat the same things, differ in the amounts consumed, their personal metabolism, their eating schedules, and even their reasons for eating.

Thus, crafting a weight loss program is an art driven by trial and error no different than sculpting except that our materials are knowledge, lifestyle choices and behavior.'

Reading 3

Excess Weight Shortens Lifespans

We all know that excess weight is bad for us. Excess weight is responsible for many early deaths. It is a precursor to hypertension, coronary heart disease, diabetes, high cholesterol, arthritis, and strokes. It also exacerbates many other conditions. Excess weight puts a burden on your internal organs as well as on the skeletal system, mainly the spine and the lower extremity joints. Excess weight in its most benign form is a source of inconvenience, discomfort and low self-esteem. In its malignant form, it threatens your wellbeing, quality of life and ultimately your very life.

Emotional suffering

Almost as bad as the physical effects of excess weight is the emotional turmoil. Emotional suffering may be one of the most painful aspects of being overweight. American society emphasizes physical appearance and often equates attractiveness with slimness, especially for women. Many people think that overweight individuals are gluttonous, lazy, or both. As a result, they often face prejudice or discrimination in the job market, at school, and in social situations. Feelings of rejection, shame, or depression are common.

The effect of excess weight on emotional well-being is important to understand. In most societies, overweight people are viewed as less desirable marriage partners, less likely to be promoted in their jobs, and tend to earn less than their more ideal-weight peers. Excess weight can also cost more. For example, many airlines now charge for two seats for an overweight person. Therefore, it is not surprising that excess weight increases the risk of major depression. In turn, depression can lead to overeating and more weight gain.

Reading 4

Physical Complications of Excess Weight

Excess weight can cause a number of physical problems that people may not be aware are attributed to excess weight. These can range from difficulties with daily activities to serious health conditions. Some of the day-to-day problems that can be caused by excess weight include breathlessness, increased sweating, and feeling excessively warm, snoring, lack of energy, joint, back, and knee problems.

Being overweight can also increase your risk of many potentially serious health conditions, including: type 2 diabetes, high blood pressure, high cholesterol, coronary heart disease, stroke, asthma, etc.

Pregnancy complications, such as gestational diabetes or pre-eclampsia (when a woman experiences a potentially dangerous rise in blood pressure during pregnancy) Most of these unpleasant conditions as a result of excess weight can be avoided by changing life-time habits and conditions that cause overeating. The point is not to resign oneself to being overweight but to take action.

Reading 5

Willpower Misunderstood

Why is it that weight loss, something so deeply desired, is so difficult to achieve? Doesn't the strength of our desire and depth of commitment translate into a large dose of willpower? The key perhaps lies in understanding willpower, knowing what it is, how it works, and how we can best use it for our purposes. Willpower is defined by the American Psychological Association as the "the ability to resist short-term temptations in order to meet long-term goals." Thus, it can be the ability to refrain from doing something we like like having a doughnut and coffee on the way to work, or it can be doing something you would rather not do, like going for a run at 4 am when you'd rather continue sleeping.

It's also a fact that willpower is limited. It is strongest in the morning but weakens as the day goes on. That is why most diets are hardest to keep during the evening. When we set goals in the form of rules and specific actions they are easier to keep. General guidelines such as; eat less carbs, stay away from refined sugars, do more exercise, etc. are difficult to follow because they are not specific. How many less carbs should you eat? Which foods have refined sugars? How much exercise is enough?

However, the rule "Don't eat after 8 pm" is clear, "Have 2 pancakes instead of your usual 3", is also clear, "walk once around the block" is also clear. You can start small; then as these goals are regularly met and as your self-control grows stronger, move on to more challenging limits. Taking on a bigger challenge than what we are ready for will just set us up for a big disappointment.

Much of the failure of losing weight hinges on our attitude towards the whole idea of weight loss. We erroneously focus our willpower on changing the type of food we eat, on doing the exercise we need to do, on counting calories, on denying ourselves certain types of food, etc. We force ourselves to comply but because we instinctively dislike changes in our routine, we can only do them for a period of time before returning to our habitual behavior.

What we can do is learn to focus our willpower on the reasons we want to lose weight such as: living longer, looking better, feeling healthier and living an overall better life. When we develop the habit of questioning whether we are eating for nutrition or for comfort, we will be on our way to planning meals, deflecting cravings, and creating habits that won't require willpower.

Another factor that contributes to the difficulty in shedding those pounds is our environment and our genetic make-up. We are subject to genetic and cultural influences that elicit the desire to eat both for survival purposes and for comfort or enjoyment. Thus, one habit worth cultivating is everytime we eat, ask ourselves if we are eating for nutrients, or for comfort.

We are setting ourselves up for failure if we do not change our mindset with respect to eating. If we understand the genetic and cultural influences that constantly urge us to eat, then we can develop personal strategies, based on vigilance and desire, to counteract both of these internal and external influences.

Weight loss means NO

People often associate weight loss with saying NO to a lot of things – **NO to pasta, NO to ice cream, NO to cake, NO to carbs.** The nature of your brain is to act upon the environment to obtain what you need. NO means STOP to the brain. The command to STOP then generates in the brain a need for a reason to stop. If you can't express the reason to yourself the commitment begins to wane. Let's look at this directive – *"Eat less carbohydrates"* The likelihood of us sticking to this command is relevant to what we know about carbohydrates. Most people don't know the differences between types and sources of carbohydrates and how they affect us. And because we are not equipped with this knowledge, we are not able to decide when it is OK to eat them and when it's not OK.

The uncertainty and confusion eventually stalls our momentum and we stop. However, if we know the differences in carbohydrates between rice, white flour, potatoes, ice cream etc., we can make decisions that will lead us in our desired direction.

Head for your ideal weight and be happy

When we understand the factors that influence our quest for weight loss, then we can see and formulate the steps that will take us to our goals. According to researchers, the experience of happiness is most intense, not when we reach our goal, but when we are engaged in the process of reaching our goal. There are three steps to reaching your goal:

1) Understand your current state,
2) Be able to see or describe your desired state,
3) Know that the steps required to get there are within your abilities.

Let's apply this to weight loss as an example.

1) You know you are overweight by 40 pounds
2) You have a photograph and memories of yourself 40 pounds lighter
3) You understand how to apply the Igen Process

Drawing from this study, the key to successful weight loss would depend on approaching it with knowledge and a can-do attitude so the motivational centers of the brain are propelled into action through the experience of "happiness" as we see the goal getting closer. Instead of focusing on the NO's, what is being "*imposed*" on us and "*deprived*" from us, we can take a positive and proactive approach and understand the concept of eating less and less in a systematic manner until we reach our desired weight. To achieve this, we must know how we personally gain weight and how our body and our mind is programmed to resist weight loss. Then and only then can we design personal strategies to achieve our goal of returning to our perfect weight. 80% of people with restrictive diets fail to continue their weight loss efforts after a period of time or they lose weight, regain it and continue their weight gain trend. A diet full of **No, Don't and Never** is doomed to fail because it is negative and prohibitive.

READING 6

The Allure of Fat, Sugar and Salt

Fat, sugar, and salt are not inherently bad. They are actually the pillars of life and health. It's the amounts we eat that make them toxic to us. It's easy to assume that all of our weight loss problems would be solved if we just eliminated fat and sugar from our diets. Unfortunately, it's not that simple. Without fat, sugar or salt, we could not live. Our body craves these substances because they are necessary to our survival. This unrestrained craving is one of the factors in our excess weight epidemic. Our body needs fat and sugar as fuel for its many internal metabolic functions as well as to maintain our musculature ready for movement. Salt is needed because it is a critical element in the various chemical reactions that take place in our body.

When we taste these substances in our food, the message we receive from our midbrain also called the limbic system is to eat as much as possible and accumulate the excess calories. It is the inadvertent and often automatic over-consumption of these substances that turn them from being beneficial to our bodies to being toxic and threatening to our organism's well-being. Our bodies need a certain number of triglycerides, cholesterol and other essential fatty acids, the scientific term for fats the body can't make on its own. These come from our food. Once the body has its immediate needs met, it will store the extra nutrients as body fat.

Fat benefits

Fats have more than twice as much energy potential (AKA calories) as do protein and carbohydrates. Specifically, fats have nine calories of energy per gram for the body, compared with four calories per gram for both carbohydrates and proteins. Fats are a vital part of the cell membrane. Without a healthy cell membrane, the rest of the cell couldn't function. They regulate the production of hormones and body temperature and form a protective cushion for your organs.

For many people this protective layer of fat may be where excess fat is being deposited first. This fat is called **visceral fat.** The body's other form of distributing fat leads to accumulating it under the skin at different points of the body and is referred to as **subcutaneous fat.** Excess visceral fat is much more dangerous since it will lead to inflammation of the affected viscera, (heart, kidneys, pancreas, etc.), because the body treats excess fat as a foreign substance.

Subcutaneous fat on the other hand, is distributed in differing patterns that are aesthetically more noticeable but are less dangerous overall (Fat may be stored on the waist first, then thighs, then abdomen, or begin in your back then neck, etc.). Usually losing weight follows this pattern in reverse by losing weight first in the last areas it was accumulated. To see if you accumulate visceral fat, lay on your back. If the excess fat flattens out over your body it is probably subcutaneous, if your gut area does not flatten and retains a mound-like shape, it is likely to be visceral fat.

Sugar benefits

Sugars, such as fructose, sucrose, or glucose are also known as carbohydrates. Our body has evolved to needing very little sugar, extracting what little it needs from its food sources. Sugar and carbohydrates are the main source of immediate energy for your body: Through the process of digestion, your body breaks down carbohydrates and converts the sugars into glucose which the cells utilize for immediate energy. An illustration of this immediate bump in energy can be readily seen when witnessing a diabetic slipping into a coma who will instantly revive upon eating a little sugar or a candy.

Salt benefits:

Salt is essential as a catalyst to many chemical reactions in our body chemistry. Sodium helps muscles and nerves work properly by assisting muscular contraction and transmission of nerve signals. Sodium also helps sustain a regular blood pH level, an important indicator of health. Furthermore, it helps to restore youthful and healthy skin. Salt regulates glucose absorption and fluid levels. It also helps to facilitate the absorption of glucose by cells, resulting in the smooth transportation of nutrients in the body's cell membranes. One of the most notable health benefits of sodium is its ability to balance the osmotic pressure in the human body due to the regulation of fluid in the body's cells.

So, as you can see, we really do need fat, sugar, and salt in our diet. To be sure that we always have these nutritional elements in our body, our brain will trigger the FTO gene to over consume these nutrients. So, it is our responsibility to regulate the body's natural tendency to overindulge, while at the same time realizing that totally eliminating these items from our diets can be bad as well.

Reading 7

Overeating, a Genetic Drive to Survive

It would seem that the title of this chapter, "Overeating, a Genetic Drive to Survive", implies that it's not your fault that you have this drive to overeat, but rather that it is something innate, inborn, that we cannot help. On the surface, this may provide some relief in that it gives you an excuse for being overweight. However, the fact that the drive to overeat is innate does not absolve you from understanding how to cope with its existence and how to deflect its harmful effects on you. But let's take a minute to look at how this all works and what we can do to use this information to our advantage.

Our Lizard Brain

Our brain's limbic system, also known as the primitive or lizard brain, is hard wired to overeat in order to maintain enough fuel reserves for times of scarcity. Not long ago in geological time, our ancestors' day was mostly spent hunting and gathering food. Their ability to store unused calories drove them to feed until full whenever there was the opportunity. They needed to prepare for times of scarcity such as winter, droughts, fires etc. So, all this worked really well for survival way back then.

Modern Times

Now here we are in the 21st century. We now have created societies where food is plentiful and easily available. Further, we also have a situation where, not only is there plenty of food, but in addition, we do not need to spend the entire day out hunting and gathering. Rather now, the majority of us spend the day in a much more sedentary way. But, in the relatively short time it has taken for our lifestyles to evolve to this modern-day ease, our brains' genetic makeup is still in scarcity mode and compelling us to overeat. And that's the problem right there!

It's in The Genes

The fairly recent discovery of the FTO gene in 2010, provided the scientific community with the culprit for the human trend toward obesity. When this gene is activated, we feel a desire to eat! However, it is also kept active by the taste of fat, sugar or salt which leads us to finishing everything on our plate and going for seconds if possible. Unfortunately, this gene is also activated by thinking about or seeing food.

The good news is that the FTO gene is an Expressive type of gene. It influences or "expresses" a specific type of behavior, in this case eating. But it does not cause eating, it merely suggests it. It is this characteristic that allows the "expression" to be stopped or modified by the cerebral cortex, our thinking brain.

We are in an evolutionary trap that leads us to accumulate fuel without an opportunity to use it!

The future, but till then...

It is likely that in the distant future, through the process of evolution, mutations will occur to adapt our brain to abundance. However, until then, it is up to us to modify this instinctual drive that leads to obesity. So, acknowledging the drive toward excess weight is key, as is developing techniques to limit eating when we have accumulated enough fuel for the day's energy requirement. Anything over the day's energy use will be stored as body fat.

Reading 8

Automatic Eating

Why Do We Eat?

Well of course, we eat because we need fuel, and the only source of immediate fuel are the fats and carbs in our food. If we don't have food, then the source of fuel is our stored body fat. But, if you are like most Americans, you know that we often eat when we are not really hungry. Sometimes it is for social reasons, sometimes it is out of boredom, but it all boils down to wanting to feel good. At the mid-brain survival level, we feel good because we are assuring ourselves of life by eating and accumulating fuel for the future.

Most eating is subconscious behavior

The drive to eat has a large instinctive and impulsive component triggered by taste, sight, smell, and recall. Eating is 70% automatic behavior. Automatic behaviors are those that occur without awareness, are initiated without intention, tend to continue without control, and operate efficiently with little or no effort.

When we begin to eat, we notice the taste, texture, aroma that tells us it's ok to continue eating. After the first few bites we become involved in the conversation or the TV program we are watching and we continue to eat without noticing taste or texture as we automatically chew, swallow, and begin on the next mouthful. The next time we consciously focus on what we are eating is when it's almost gone or when we are so full it becomes uncomfortable to eat.

Hunger has nothing to do with it

Having easy access to abundant food, Many people in this society have difficulty remembering or even knowing what true hunger feels like. Most often, eating is triggered by our desire for comfort or joy. If you find yourself reaching for that cookie or bag of chips, even though you have just eaten, then most definitely hunger is not the reason. In many instances, the greatest craving to eat happens during times of emotional turmoil – during times of sadness or great stress. Common triggers include unemployment, concerns about finances, relationship issues, work related stress and a whole spectrum of other emotional reasons.

Eating forces a good feeling on you which is great. However, the good feeling goes away as soon as you swallow. To renew the good feeling, we need to take another bite or spoonful and there we are on a merry-go-round. We eat because it's time to eat. It fills a void when there is nothing else to do, or because it's just there.

Food, a feel-good source

Eating can be triggered as well by happiness and satisfaction as when you're celebrating an accomplishment or when there is a special occasion. When we feel good we want to feel even better and eating always raises the pleasure and happiness level. In other words, your brain will prompt you to eat in a variety of circumstances that are totally unrelated to hunger.

So, What Can Be Done?

The urge to eat may become so automatic that it feels like it cannot be controlled. But in truth, it is a learned response developed over the years. You can become aware of those automatic desires and urges and develop strategies that rely on your reasoning abilities to deal with them and counteract their influences. Rest assured it does not happen overnight, but knowing you are in control and know how to handle these automatic urges is a huge step forward.

Reading 9

The Mathematics of Weight Gain and Weight Loss

Getting started on a weight reducing program can be daunting if you don't know where and how to start. Resolve is one thing, but it is all totally wasted if there is no clear path, no road map or benchmarks guiding you towards your goal of losing weight.

What you eat counts

Consuming more calories in a day than you use up in that day will make you gain weight. This is basic physiology. Conversely, consuming less calories than you are burning in a day will make you lose weight.

Many other factors will also affect the results of calorie intake needed such as sex, age, lifestyle, activity level, type of food eaten, metabolic rate, and overall general health. A 25-year-old six-foot male who regularly goes to the gym will understandably need more calories than a five-foot 70-year-old grandma – unless of course grandma is into extreme sports and goes biking and rock climbing every other day With all these factors taken into consideration, the amount of food eaten is the single largest predictor of obesity.

This places the solution within reach of any normal healthy person. Finding out how many calories it takes to maintain your weight or to gain weight will give an insight into how to modify your intake to begin your weight loss process.

Not rocket science

This information is not rocket science. We would like a magic bullet, that pill, or drink, or food, that will let us ignore that amount is relevant and lose weight anyway, but it just does not exist. However, you can work with your brain, your habits, your subconscious, your triggers, to put you in control once and for all.

Most of us live far more sedentary lives now than we did when we were 16 and "could eat anything." So, take an honest look at yourself, take the food survey, and this will give you a starting point. Eat a little less than you need to stay at the weight you are, and you are on that road to shedding those unwanted pounds. How much less? The recommendation is to reduce your daily calorie intake by 500 calories to lose 1 to 2 pounds a week.

Or you can take off 10% off your average daily intake and see how much weight comes off. These recommendations are just starting points and everything depends on how much weight you want to lose, the type of exercise you are doing (or not), the type of diet you are eating and your metabolism. Not everyone is the same and you need to determine for yourself which formula works for you.

Let me say that again. Everyone is different and you need to choose a combination of strategies you think will work the best for you in the long term. Trial and error will determine which strategies work best for you so you can incorporate them into your lifestyle. And in working with you, we ensure that you come up with an individualized program you can follow because it is in sync with your lifestyle.

Reading 10

The Use of Imagery and Affirmations

Close your eyes and imagine yourself at your perfect weight at the beach. Imagine yourself walking on the beach with the sand warm on your feet, the sun bright in your eyes, the breeze softly blowing... Now picture yourself at your perfect weight standing in front of an inviting spot and seeing a hammock. Imagine yourself climbing into the hammock and swinging gently under the shade of tropical palms feeling so relaxed that you find yourself getting sleepy.

I am sure at some point in your life, you have undergone this experiment and actually felt yourself being transported to some tropical island and lulled into a state of relaxation. Ever wonder how this is so? Studies show that the areas stimulated in the brain during times of imagination and actual perception seem to be similar. During real experiences, our neocortex or reasoning brain receives information from the senses that constitute our sense of reality.

However, when reality is disconnected, as when we sleep, the experience of a dream becomes as real as if it were happening while you were awake. Think of the times that you have had a nightmare and you wake up sweaty, heart beating wildly convinced that there was a hooded person with fiery eyes chasing you. The relief of engaging your physical senses again and realizing it was just a dream comforts you. It is this characteristic of the brain, the inability to distinguish fantasy from reality, that gives the use of imagery and affirmations their power.

What is imagery?

According to the *Stanford Encyclopedia of Psychology,* Mental imagery such as "visualizing," "seeing in the mind's eye," "imagining the feel of," etc.) are quasi-perceptual experiences they resemble perceptual experience, but occur in the absence of the appropriate external stimuli

What is an affirmation?

In contrast, affirmation is the attempt to create new thought habits. It is a positive thought that you choose to adopt into your belief system to produce a specific desired result. The simplest form of affirmation involves repeating a new idea about yourself to yourself on a regular basis.

This exercise is used in a variety of situations. It is most commonly used to increase self-esteem or to motivate people to perform certain actions. Noted French hypnotherapist Emile Coue (1857-1926) discovered that if you repeat an affirmation often enough the brain will begin to adopt the belief.

Application of imagery and affirmation.

Because of their very nature, imagery and affirmation are effective weapons in your weight loss arsenal. For example, you may take a photograph of yourself, at your current weight and affix it next to a picture of a younger and leaner you. This will give direction to your actions motivating you to continue with what you are doing. The more you look at the two images, the more you become accustomed to the image you want. Once you begin to use images and affirmative phrases in your weight loss plan, they lodge into your subconscious as potential realities. The more you "see" them, the more they begin to exert a subliminal effect on your behavior.

In sports, mental practice is common among athletes. They see themselves throwing, catching, or swinging knowing that it translates into expertise. When an athlete actually throws, catches or swings, the brain is involved directing muscles and posture etc. It stands to reason that if you visualize an action, there must be a subliminal effect on the muscles also.

Reading 11

Becoming an Expert

We all want to achieve goals in our lives — optimum health, a successful business, recognition, quitting smoking, and so on. Becoming an expert is the end result of immersing yourself in a specific area. One measure is if you spend 10,000 hours on a subject you will become an expert in that subject. However, expertise is relative, you know more than some and you know less than others. Becoming an expert on a particular subject is having less people know more than you and knowing more than most people.

Expert secrets

There are no secrets or shortcuts to becoming an expert. We already know from what we've read or observed from successful people, it takes hard work, focus and dedication at a minimum. A passion to succeed is a very helpful attribute as well. And keeping one's eye on the goal. The good thing is, once one has become an expert at something, mastered it, the feeling of accomplishment is amazing. And it also gives us the courage to undertake the next task, project, hurdle, etc., thus increasing our expertise.

Making new behavior automatic

Researchers found that it takes more than two months before a new behavior becomes automatic. How long it takes each of us individually to form a new habit can vary depending on the strength of previous habits, your social environment, and family support. It has taken a lifetime to get to where you are. However, in a fraction of that time you can reverse your weight gain. But you must first become an expert on your eating behavior and understand how you gain weight. Only then can you devise strategies rooted in a solid base of knowledge.

Reading 12

Food Combinations That Affect Your Metabolic Rate

We often hear that having a fast metabolic rate is a good thing when trying to manage weight, but what exactly does this mean and more importantly what can you do to increase your metabolic rate?

What is metabolism?

Metabolism is a set of life sustaining chemical reactions our body performs to convert food into energy, to enable digestion, to repair cells, etc. Food that is not converted into immediate energy is stored as body fat. The speed of a person's metabolism affects his body's absorptions of nutrients. A slow metabolism will increase absorption while a fast metabolism decreases it. The pace of this process varies from person to person and is affected by many factors.

Some factors that affect the metabolic rate are:

- Height and weight, the larger a person is, the faster is his metabolism.

- A lean body mass and a high activity level will elicit a faster metabolism.

How your diet can speed up your metabolism

As mentioned above, the rate of a person's metabolism affects the body's absorption of nutrients. It is also affected by the combination of foods a person eats. Meals can be categorized by the percentage of protein, fat and carbohydrates contained in the mix. If 60% or more of the nutrients are derived from carbohydrates your metabolism will slow down. On the other hand, if 60% or more are proteins and/or fats, your metabolic rate will speed up. A faster metabolism will burn more calories per minute while reducing the amount of time nutrients are in your body.

Reading 13

Malleability of Food Preferences

We are an adaptive species. We manipulate our physical environment as well as our mental environment to create comfort or be in harmony with the outside world. Our limbic system, also referred to as the lizard brain or primitive brain, adapts to an environment that guarantees the survival of the organism. The mechanism that enables this adaptation is called **"neural plasticity"**. It allows for brain cells to acquire new functions as needed, and to discard previous functions. For example, a three-month abstinence from a highly-preferred food will dampen and eventually eliminate the brain's desire for that specific food. It adapts to the absence! Even if you know that the specific food is in the shelves of your market or even your pantry, as long as you don't eat it, the brain will begin to habituate to its absence.

Conversely, eating food that is disliked will be tolerated at first and with continued use eventually a preference will develop. It is within your abilities to discover, develop and use this adaptive ability as needed.

Childhood has a big influence in food preferences

The development of children's food preferences is influenced by genetic, familial, and environmental factors. There have been studies showing strong genetic influence on appetite in children, but the environment also plays an important role in shaping children's eating preferences. High-fat and sweet foods are usually preferred by infants and children in many countries, even across species, whereas vegetables are almost universally rejected.

This is proof of our genetic impulse to prefer high calorie foods. Had there not been any meat or milk, the vegetables would have been chosen. Indeed, our species up to this century has been primarily vegetarian. While male hunters occasionally brought meat to the table, there were always vegetables, tubers, roots, and fruits gathered by the women. Also, introducing variety to your children at an early age opens them up to be willing to and wanting to experience new meals during their entire lifetimes

There is evidence that the food environment that parents create at home shapes children's food preferences and food acceptance patterns, such that availability and exposure to foods can affect children's food selections and intake.

The good news is that you can condition yourself to like things. Most people have to train themselves to enjoy a new kind of diet when a lifestyle change is needed for medical reasons. For example, if you stop adding salt to your food, then after a few appallingly bland and colorless weeks, your palate will become more sensitive to other tastes, and you'll be able to get by with less salt. The preference for a particular taste or the drive to have a particular taste can both vary significantly over time.

In any case, perception and prejudice influence taste although it is almost impossible to separate the sensory experience from the suggestion of the subconscious. These things become self-fulfilling:

like the infant wailing over the broccoli, the more you tell yourself you don't like something, the more vile it seems. Have you ever had to train yourself to like something? Are there any foods you used to love that you can no longer eat?

And is it worth trying to enjoy them again? You must always remember that you are in control and you can change not only your behavior but your food preferences, likes, and dislikes.

Reading 14

How to Deal with Cravings

Cravings don't just occur when you see or smell a specific food. They are also aroused when you hear about it, or think about it! In fact, the craving may start at some point in time before you become conscious of the desire. The process is as follows; as you drive you see a billboard for a sports car and you turn your attention back to the road. However, your mind registers the scene, a tailgate party before a football game where they are grilling meat. This reminds you of your football game party a couple of months ago, and you remember the spicy hamburger patties your uncle brought and how tasty they were. A few minutes later as you pass a fast food outlet, you feel hungry for a hamburger and you pull in.

What just happened? Technically, your brain was hijacked by the midbrain. The moment you saw the billboard and the grilled meat, a subconscious reaction began. Cells tuned into salient stimuli fired as they saw the chicken. These sent a signal to cells in the reward center, in effect alerting them to the possibility of a pleasure event, then the reward center cells invite you to eat by sending a conscious thought to the cerebral cortex urging you to think "I'm hungry."

Trick your brain

However, the craving begins, as soon as you become aware of the craving, you have a short window of time to act. If you vacillate you lose! To successfully deny a craving, **first** acknowledge the pleasure of yielding to the temptation by saying "eating this would be so good and would taste great." **Then,** recite the cons of yielding to the temptation such as, "it will derail my progress", "I will regret it" I can get it later" etc., **and finally,** engage your mind in thinking of a real issue that you are dealing with in your personal life or at work; your children, your business, your elderly parents, the planned remodeling etc. The premise is that you can't have two thoughts at the same time. As soon as you stop thinking about the potential pleasure, the craving will subside and release its hold on you.

Why Do We Crave Sugar?

According to Christine Gerbstadt, MD, RD, a dietitian and American Dietetic Association (ADA) spokeswoman, "Sweet is the first taste humans prefer from birth." Carbohydrates stimulate the release of feel-good brain chemicals that calm and relax us, and offer a natural "high," says Susan Moores, MS, RD, Sugar is a carbohydrate, but carbohydrates come in other forms, too, such as whole grains, fruits, and vegetables. Sweets just taste good, too. With all that going for it, why wouldn't we crave sugar?

When you're under stress, your body releases the hormone cortisol, which signals your brain to seek out rewards. Comfort foods loaded with sugar and fat are an immediate source of pleasure. When you reach for food to mitigate or allay negative feelings such as frustration, anger or sadness, you inadvertently create a powerful association in your brain between food and feeling good.

If your cravings start to run amok and demand satisfaction every day, take heart: You're not at the mercy of your food desires. You can learn to outsmart them. What you need is a plan that stops this natural cycle. Not all of the following work for everyone so it's up to you to find among these strategies those with which you are comfortable.

Strategies to Break the Craving Cycle

1. Eat a bit of what you're craving, maybe a small cookie or a fun size candy bar, suggests Kerry Neville, MS, RD, a registered dietitian and ADA spokeswoman. Enjoying a little of what you love can help you steer clear of feeling denied. You can indulge in it, but just do it less frequently. Plan ways to enjoy your favorite foods in controlled portions, says McManus. Get a slice of pizza instead of a whole pie, or share a piece of restaurant cheesecake with two friends. Before you dig in, dole out a small amount of the food you want (on a plate) and put the rest away
2. Don't substitute food cravings. Trying to quell a food craving with a low-cal imitation won't satisfy your brain's memory center, says Marcia Levin Pelchat, PhD, If you're craving a milkshake, yogurt won't cut it. Munching five crackers, a handful of popcorn, and a bag of pretzels, all in the name of trying to squash a craving for potato chips, will net you more calories than if you'd eaten a single serving bag.
3. Combine craved foods with healthy ones. You can still fill yourself up and satisfy a sugar craving, too. For example, if you crave chocolate you can dip a banana in chocolate sauce or mix some almonds with chocolate chips.
4. Reach for fruit. Keep fruit handy for when sugar cravings hit. You'll get fiber and nutrients along with some sweetness. And stock up on foods like nuts, seeds, and dried fruits, says certified addiction specialist Judy Chambers, LCSW, CAS. Have them handy so you reach for them instead of reaching for the old sugary treat.

5. Get up and go. When a sugar craving hits, take a walk around the block or do something to change the scenery, to take your mind off the food you're craving. Distract yourself with a non-food-related activity until the craving goes away. It could be walking the dog or doing push ups or calling a friend.

You may need more than one strategy to thwart sugar cravings. Mix it up. One week you may find success with one tactic, and another week calls for an alternative approach. What's important is to "have a 'bag of tricks' to try, to tame sugar cravings, you really need to figure out what works for you. Lastly, go easy on yourself but keep your goals in mind!

Reading 15

Setting up your own Igen Process center:

Let us certify you to deliver the Igen Process

Receive materials and support to form groups in your community

Contact us at The Igen Process, 6507 Issac Ct. Chino, California 91710

the-art-of-weight-reduction.com

Biography

I spent the last 36 years in the Los Angeles Unified School District's Adult Education Division. Upon retiring in 2010, I weighed 250 pounds. This was 110 pounds over my first years on the job in 1976. And this was after many bouts of yoyo dieting in the intervening years. I am now only 30 pounds away from my ideal weight of 140 which I will gradually reach in the near future through the process I have created. Much of my insight in developing the Igen Process came after reading Dr. Kessler's book, "The end of overeating", a seminal look at the physiology of weight. It was after reading his research that I shifted my focus from weight loss to weight gain. This led me eventually to formalize the Igen Process as a behavioral approach to weight reduction that allows you to bypass exercise and diet in reaching your ideal weight.

www.ingramcontent.com/pod-product-compliance
Lightning Source LLC
LaVergne TN
LVHW040159080526
838202LV00042B/3238